SEX SECRETS

FOR MEN

69

SEX SECRETS WOMEN WISH YOU KNEW BUT WILL NEVER TELL YOU

This book was published thanks to free support and training from:

DigitalBiz.com.ng

TABLE OF CONTENTS

INTRODUCTION

Hello! I'm glad you have taken the time to purchase this book. I intended it to be the **perfect book to sex secrets**, ideal whether you're a beginner or an experienced lover. This book should give you **all the tools you need** to completely satisfy your lover.

Inside you'll learn:

- How to spice up your sex life and a hero to your woman
- My favorite sex and relationship tips
- Everything you need to know about how to satisfy your woman
- ...and full, total disclosure on over 60 sex secrets!

Let's face it: No matter how proficient you think you are, every now and then, you could use a little boost to improve your sex life and satisfy your partner. Try these simple, achievable sex tips with your lover tonight.

Want to have even better sex for a very long time? You've been handed a right book, my friend.

It's taken me a long time to bring this information together, but I think it was worth the effort.

So here it is – the **most important** things I've learned about sex from my own experiences and the experiences of my friends. It's frank, it's eye-opening, and it may surprise and shock you. But it's all true.

Here are our 65 best sex secrets and relationship tips. Don't worry, you can thank me later. So why is this sex secret important? And what do you need to know to master those secrets? Read on!

I very much hope that this information helps you to become a masterful lover.

Warmest regards,
Babalola Wasiu

THE SEX SECRETS

1. Give Her Sexy Thoughts

According to the *Journal of Sex and Marital Therapy*, researcher Rosemary Basson, MD concludes that women must convince themselves to want sex before their sexual desire kicks in. Arousal starts first in the mind. Give your woman sexy thoughts throughout the day to stir her sexual desire.

Send her sexy text messages or emails while she's at work. Include little reminders from when you had great sex. Tell her what you want to do to her once she gets home. If your hesitant and are afraid she'll be offended, start off with a fun flirty text message. You'll hot text messages such as "I love every bone in your body, including mine!" These sexy messages are just what shc needs to start thinking about sex and becoming aroused throughout my day.

2. Come Home Dirty and Sweaty

Believe it or not, women love rugged looking men. There's something secretly sexy about dirty men. Brad Pitt, Harrison Ford, and Russell Crowe for instance, are irresistible to women because of their renegade appearance. Not only that, the scent of sweat is an aphrodisiac to women.

According to James V. Kohl, coauthor of "The Scent of Eros," women are led by their sense of smell when it comes to sexual attraction. They are especially receptive at detecting pheromones, a special aromatic chemical released by humans to sexually attract one another. Another study, conducted by Bern University known as the "Stinky T-shirt Study" concluded that women were attracted to the pheromone chemicals left behind by men's sweat.

3. Talk about sex.

As time passes in a relationship, it's easy to get into a rut and just go through the motions, rather than express what you really want (and need) in bed. Sex therapist Williams Lucena, FMD, says it's time to break this cycle with some frank talk. "Ask each other, 'What do I need in bed from you?'" he suggests. "Get back to the communication you used to have."

4. Kegels, Kegels, Kegels.

For those of you who refuse to go to the gym, you're in luck – there is a sex specific exercise that you can perform anywhere, any time. And it won't make you sweat.

The kegel exercise is the rhythmic clenching and relaxing of the pubococcygeal muscle (usually abbreviated as PC muscle, though it has nothing to do with political correctness).

The PC muscle is directly related to sexual satisfaction for both men and women.

If you want to last longer during sex, you're not alone. "Premature ejaculation is a problem that affects almost every man at some point in his life," Thomas J. Walsh, M.D., an urologist at the University of Washington, told us.

One way to delay ejaculation is by doing kegels. Strengthening the pubococcygeal (PC) muscles of the pelvic floor will help you control your orgasms during sex.

5. Experiment with edging.

Another way to make sex last longer? Train yourself to delay your orgasm while you're masturbating. Edging — the act of bringing yourself to the brink of orgasm and then stopping all sexual stimulation — is a common technique for avoiding premature ejaculation.

6. Try a vibrator.

Lots of guys enjoy a vibrating sensation on their penis — particularly around the frenulum. A 2012 study found that 44% of heterosexual dudes have enjoyed using a vibrator at some point.

Vibrators have long been marketed to and used by women, but that's changing. The Tenuto from MysteryVibe, for instance, is a small vibrating clip that attaches to the base of your penis; you can use it on your own or during intercourse.

7. Let her take the lead.

Men so often take the lead in bed. Sometimes, the key to better sex is letting her be in charge. "Don't be afraid to let your mate lead," says Joyce Morley, EdD, a licensed counselor in Decatur, Ga. "Allow your mate to initiate sexual pleasure on occasions, as well as taking the top position."

8. Plan a memorable first date

Your crush has probably been on a million and one coffee dates, so consider planning something more unique — like a trip to the farmer's market followed by a picnic, a visit to the aquarium, or a pottery class.

9. Find a condom that feels great..

If you hate the way condoms make you feel during sex, you might not be wearing the right ones, according to sex therapist Ian Kerner, Ph.D., author of *She Comes First: The Thinking Man's Guide to Pleasuring a Woman*. When picking a condom, find one that fits like a glove, and look for rubbers that are ribbed or ultra-thin.

Condoms are highly effective at preventing pregnancy and STIs, so it's worth finding the one that feels best for you.

10.   Eat healthy.

This doesn't sound like a sex tip, but treating your body right with good nutrition helps the whole body, including your libido, says Debbie Mandel, a stress management expert and author of *Addicted to Stress*. "Eat healthy foods to reduce cholesterol and keep your cardiovascular system humming," she adds. "This will ensure that circulation is at peak performance for the 'southern hemisphere.'"

11.   Do your household chores.

Want to put your wife in the mood for better sex? "Help around the house," says Mandel. "The best foreplay happens outside the bedroom. By helping with chores and errands, you make them feel valued."

12.   Do it standing up.

We promise — it isn't as complicated as it seems.

Start by standing against the wall with your partner facing you and straddling one of your legs — it'll make it easier for them balance, according to sexologist Eric Marlowe Garrison, author of *Mastering Multiple Position Sex.*

13.   Make love instead.

Does it feel lately like it's just sex? "Try *making love,*" advises Dr. Morley. "You make love with that special someone, but you have sex with anybody."

14.   Try prostate massage.

The prostate is a walnut-sized gland located between the bladder and rectum, and it contains tons of nerve endings. Stimulating the prostate can feel so good, some sexual health experts have dubbed it the "male G-spot."

15.   Lube up.

According to Bencivenga, there's no shame in using lubricant to satisfy women. "Many guys think that since women get wet, if we aren't wet, then we aren't into it," she says. "That's not true. Sometimes, whether it's stress, certain times of the month, or fatigue, women can have a hard time getting physically aroused even when they are mentally in the game. Lubricant in the bedside drawer is your new best friend."

Lubrication increases the comfort and speed with which you can penetrate the vagina and grind against the clitoris," Ellen Friedrichs, M.A., an adjunct professor of human sexuality at Rutgers University, says "But sometimes, no matter how turned on a woman might be psychologically, she can have trouble getting wet."

That's where lube comes in. Try squeezing a few drops onto the tip of your penis before you start intercourse.

16.   Use Blindfolds

Focusing on the senses is extremely arousing. Blindfolds are a great way for women to focus on his every touch and for men to learn exactly what pleases his women.

17.   Practice self-care.

"Take good care of your penis," says Dr. Simmons. "Penile injury is usually sustained when your partner is on top or when the penis buckles from missed penetration. If things are getting out of hand, ask your partner to ease up. If you suspect a penile fracture due to a perceived 'pop' followed by bruising, see a urologist immediately."

18.   Don't forget foreplay.

Regardless of how you get revved up for better sex, Matthew N. Simmons, MD, PhD, of the Glickman Urological and Kidney Institute in Cleveland, suggests not skimping on the foreplay no matter how long you have been together as a couple. "Foreplay contributes greatly to stronger orgasms and improved sex," he says. "Gearing up your autonomic nervous system will increase sensitivity, excitement, and strength of orgasm. Your patience and attentiveness will pay dividends."

Sex isn't a race. Take time to explore your partner before you get to intercourse. Not only will it build desire, but it'll help you discover what you and your partner do and don't like in bed.

"On its own, sex is pretty mechanical," psychologist and relationship therapist Tracy Thomas, Ph.D., says "Foreplay is where you learn what you like and don't like."

19. Change up the stimulation

When you're all the way inside her, add side-to-side movement or up-and-down pelvic pressure against her clitoris to vary the stimulation.

20.   Make a fantasy lottery.

Both you and your partner write five sexual fantasies down on five separate notebook cards. Then head to a restaurant where you can get a booth and some privacy in a public setting.

Over dinner and wine, pull out the cards and make three piles: "yes"; "maybe someday"; and "not on your life." Put the items from the first two piles in a shoe box, and once a month — or as often as you like — pull one out to try.

21.   Exercise.

Few things will get you ready to satisfy women quite like getting in regular exercise each day, says Matthew N. Simmons, MD, PhD, of the Glickman Urological and Kidney Institute in Cleveland. "Even as little as 15 minutes of exercise daily will improve self-esteem, self-image, and libido," he says. "Exercise makes the physical aspects of sex more enjoyable. Furthermore, making exercise a habit promotes cardiovascular health, which is necessary for normal erectile function."

22.   But don't overdo it.

Too much exercise can have the opposite effect, says Pete McCall, MS, an exercise physiologist with the American Council on Exercise. "Being in an overtraining state produces general feelings of fatigue and low energy and can disrupt sleep patterns and change mood," he says. "This is hardly a good combination for wooing a romantic partner."

23.   Exercise together.

Think of it as fat-burning foreplay. Exercise will raise your dopamine levels and ease your anxiety. Bonus: Your post-run sweat has androstadienone, a testosterone derivative that can spike your partner's arousal when they smell it. So, exercising with your lover is an even better sex tip, says Mandel. "Working out together ensures that both libidos and endorphins will be up," she says. "Since you're both already sweating, take it to the next level. Stretching together is also a good idea."

24.   Use your tongue wisely.

When kissing, don't use your tongue like a dart (in and out, in and out). Instead, try varying motions and amounts of pressure.

25.   Take her Dancing

Many men aren't aware of the **sexuality in dancing**. While, romantic dinners can lead to the bedroom there is nothing more arousing than a night out dancing. When women are dancing, they begin to think of their body as sexy and graceful. Their self confidence increases and are no longer shy to expose it later on during the night. Dancing is like an ego booster for women. A woman can let loose, dress sexy, and feel good about herself. Not

to mention, the atmosphere in a club, is less intimidating and proper than a fancy restaurant. I'm not saying to

skip the fancy restaurant; in fact it's crucial to show women that they deserve to be treated with respect and class.

However, a night of dancing helps **jump start the sexual chemistry** between two people.

26.   Make circles on her clitoris.

An Indiana University survey of 1,055 women found that 3 out of 4 women like it when you trace circles on her clitoris with your fingers or tongue. If you're not sure what drives your partner wild, ask her!

27.   Be wary of constant direct clitoral contact.

The clitoris is packed with nerves and super sensitive, so your partner may not want you to touch her there directly.

The clitoris actually extends several inches under the skin on either side of her vagina — like a wishbone — which means you can massage it without applying direct pressure. Trace the extensions with flat, wide, extra-wet tongue strokes, or slow finger zigzags (don't forget lube). Then rub a slow spiral around the top, drawing closer with each pass. The combination of anticipation and indirect contact will bring her pleasure centers to life.

28.   Do doggy-style the right way.

Doggy-style tip: For over-the-top stimulation of her most nerve-packed parts, keep doing

short and shallow thrusts, rather than deep
and fast ones.

29.   Quit smoking.

There are a lot of benefits to quitting smoking
— and one of them is better sex. There's
evidence that smoking can affect the size and
strength of your erection, and that smokers
may have smaller penises than nonsmokers.

"In addition to damaging blood vessels,
smoking may cause damage to penile tissue
itself, making it less elastic and preventing it
from stretching."

**30.   Hang out with your married
pals.**

Looking for the right person? Don't abandon
your married or coupled-up friends. A guy
with a spouse or live-in partner has an
expanded social circle — meaning he knows
more eligible bachelors and bachelorettes

(that he could potentially introduce you to) than he did when he was single.

31.   Send her a letter.

The art of letter-writing is definitely underrated. Write your partner one that does not involve a laser printer or an e-mail address. Write what you feel, but the ruling sentiment should be one of gratitude and confidence in your future together. Then mail it to them.

32.   "V" is for victory.

To increase clitoral contact when a woman's on top, make a V with two fingers, and place it so the point of the V (just between the two knuckles) is directly over her clitoris. Your fingers should come down on either side of your penis as she rides you. This will stimulate the clitoris, inner labia, and urethra — as well as add intensity for you.

33.   Call within 48 hours.

Forget the rules: if an attractive person gives you their number; call or text within 48 hours. Otherwise, you'll look like you're scared — or just stupid for resorting to juvenile mind games.

34.   Leave a confident voicemail.

Yes, it's a little old school, but if you get their voicemail, leave a message. To convey confidence, your voice should be deep and moderately loud. Stand up and hum a little before you call — it will bring your voice to the ideal pitch.

35.   Don't immediately head south during foreplay.

During foreplay, the genitals are off-limits. Touch the other parts of your partner's body, using fingers, a feather, a silk scarf, or anything that turns them on — and ask them to describe how it feels. This builds the tension until you're both ready to explode.

36.   Abstain a bit.

Believe it or not, it's a surefire way to improve sex and make your next encounter with your lover even more exciting. "Practice abstinence for a couple of days, a weekend, or a week," says Mandel. "Abstinence does make the heart grow fonder and makes you lust after forbidden fruit."

37.   Ease into dirty talk.

Want to know if your partner likes to talk dirty? Say something like, "You make me think dirty thoughts." Ease in slowly. It's best to test the waters a bit, rather than immediately go for your deepest, kinkiest dirty talk right off the bat.

38.   Don't ignore the perineum.

Stimulating the perineum — the area between your balls and your butt — can feel really good during masturbation or sex. "This area is packed with nerve-endings, so it feels really sensitive". You can also ask your partner to apply pressure to the area during oral sex.

39.   Shop for new cologne.

If you don't have cologne that your partner likes, shop for something new together. It's a form of foreplay. (We like Jimmy Choo Man Eau de Toilette, $110

40.   Hold hands.

It sounds simple, but holding hands can work as an aphrodisiac. It shows your partner you're devoted, and proud to tell the world.

41.   Try it on the washing machine.

Everyone wants to try sex standing up, but not everyone has the physical strength to pull it off.

Here's an easier alternative from our guide to extreme sex positions: Have your partner sit on a sturdy, high-up surface — like a desk or a washing machine — and wrap their legs around your body. Enjoy!

42.   Focus on relaxation.

Men like to get excited for better sex, but women are more likely to get in the mood through relaxation. "Wash her hair in the shower or massage her scalp to relax her," says Debbie Mandel, a stress management expert and author of *Addicted to Stress*. "A woman needs to be relaxed before she is ready to receive."

43.   Praise your partner.

Compliment your mate in front of your friends; it shows you're proud to have them as your partner.

44.   Boost your testosterone.

Research shows that when you have more testosterone in your bloodstream, your orgasms are more frequent — and more powerful. Here's how to know if your T levels are low — and, if that's the case, how to give them a much-needed boost.

45.   Show passion.

"Passion" means being in the moment and not being distracted. Sex is a conversation, and your partner doesn't want to feel like you wish you had your iPhone.

46. Whisper your fantasies in public.

Lie on a blanket in a park, and whisper fantasies to one another, sparing no detail. You'll create sexual tension — but with safety, as there's no possibility of sex then and there.

47. Create anticipation.

Use anticipation as an aphrodisiac. Instead of tearing their clothes off, take your time. Tell them what you want to do with each section of their exposed skin.

48. Make use of technology.

Want to keep her in the mood for sex later that night while you're stuck at the office? Use your cell phone or e-mail. "Send her sexy messages throughout the day," advises Mandel.

49.   Don't neglect the neck.

The neck is super-sensitive, and it's one of the sexiest places to stimulate your partner during foreplay or intercourse. We recommend trailing your lips from her collarbone to her jaw, then gently kissing her neck.

50.   When you're on a date, sit at a 90-degree angle, not across from your partner.

When you're out for dinner, always position yourself at a 90-degree angle to your date rather than straight on. If your date sits at the end of the table, sit in the first seat to their left. Turn toward them from the waist, which will give the person the opportunity to turn toward you.

51.   Never agree to disagree.

When you and your partner fight, never agree to disagree. Agreeing to disagree shuts down the communication process and resolves nothing. And the less comfortable your other half feels about communicating with you, the less confident they'll feel about the relationship.

52.   Ask her for a kissing lesson.

Ask her to demonstrate what she considers a sexy kiss. Then let her do all the work. It's educational...and fun.

53.   Mix things up in bed.

If you're experiencing a case of the "same-old, same-old," working on adding a little variety is the key to better sex, says Simmons. "Spice things up by planning and discussing variations on your usual sexual habits," he explains, "Don't be afraid to mix things up in bed, whether it's a pair of fuzzy handcuffs, toys, new positions, and other creative additions can enhance intimacy and orgasm." Sexual novelty re-creates those early-relationship, take-me-now hormones.

54.   Plan for sex.

It may not sound that romantic, but Dr. Simmons says it's a great way to improve your sex life and satisfy women. Construct a plan for having sex, he suggests: "Setting aside time or arranging opportunities for sex is very important, especially for busy couples or those with children. Don't let the frequency of sex dwindle due to fatigue or the inability to find the 'right time.'"

55.   Fund a sexy shopping spree.

Write out a gift certificate with an expiration date that coincides with your evening at a hotel. If she prefers to shop alone, let her—either way, you'll find out what interests her.

56.   Start volunteering.

Join a volunteer group. Selflessness is sexy—and research has shown that women consider altruism more important than men do

57.   Have sex in a new place.

Start sex outside the bedroom. The same old place leads to the same old patterns. So explore some new erogenous areas: The kitchen. The bathroom. Your bodies will be in new places, making it unlikely that you'll follow old routines.

58.   Use touch even without sex.

Even when you're not having sex, you can still improve your sex life by using touch in an intimate, but not sexual, way. "Touching is important, but doesn't always mean sex," says Morley. "It is important to be intimate with your mate by touching her with love and affection on a daily basis. Kiss daily, and don't be afraid to allow her to reciprocate."

59.   Do yoga.

Yoga has plenty of benefits for men —
including improving your sex life.

"Because yoga helps people develop a sense of calmness, strength, stamina, agility, knowledge of their own bodies, and the ability to remain in the present moment and make small adjustments, it can greatly enhance sexual performance and confidence," says sex therapist Gracie Landes, LMFT, CST.

Research shows that practicing an hour of yoga every day is linked to delaying ejaculation and boosting your overall sexual performance. It can also help work those all-important pelvic floor muscles.

60.   Don't ask your partner if she finished.

Here's something you should never ask a woman after sex: "Did you come?"

By posing that question *after* sex, rather than during the act itself, you're implicitly telling your partner that their pleasure is an afterthought for you — and that's not okay. Instead, make her pleasure a priority during sex itself.

61.   Use your old college beanbag chair for a new purpose.

Here's a new place to have sex: in a beanbag chair. You can contour it to any shape, and it'll support you in unexpected ways.

62.   Think like a woman.

Natalie Bencivenga, co-founder, editor, and writer of twodaymag.com, advises thinking like a woman. "To think like a woman in bed, you don't have to be one," she says. "Give attention to some of her most neglected areas, like her neck, her feet, her inner thighs. Tease her mercilessly. Make her want it. You will be surprised what a build-up will bring!"

63.   Have sex in a forest.

Pitch your tent in a national park like Alaska's Denali National Park, where 6 million untamed acres and a crowd-thinning permit system leave little risk of waking the neighbors. Your partner will gasp when the midnight sun bathes Mt. McKinley in salmon pink light.

64.   Compliment her body.

Want a foolproof way to drive her wild and ensure better sex? "Find a particular feature, and tell her that she is the best in this class," says Mandel.

65.   Watch porn together.

We'll let you in on a little secret: lots of women *love* watching porn. According to a survey, 75% of women said they were down to watch porn with a partner during foreplay or sex itself. That said, they may not be into the same type of content you're into, so be sure to discuss your tastes beforehand or scope out some softer-core fare. (Director Erika Lust's LustFilms is a great place to start.)

66. Fool around in the backseat of a car.

Take your partner to the garage and reclaim a space you long ago ceded: the backseat of the car. There's a throwback, high school quality to it that'll turn both of you on.

67. Earn your right to experiment.

Sexual experimentation is earned, not inherited. It requires time, tact, and trust: 66 percent of the women we surveyed said they're most willing to experiment later in a relationship.

68. Give her a proper warm-up

Clitoral contact in particular feels abrasive without a proper warm-up. If a woman yips or inhales suddenly when you go there — instead of purring or moaning — you've jumped the gun.

69.   Try the Fusion

Try the sex position known as the "Fusion":
You both sit up and she faces you, sitting on
your lap so she can lift her legs onto your
shoulders. This increases the muscular
tension that advances the orgasm sequence.
By elevating her butt off the bed, it'll be easier
for her to thrust and grind in circles.

CONCLUSION

Now that you've read this book, the most important thing you can do is put this information to work for you. The best advice I can give you is, don't try to do everything at once. Introduce new sexual techniques slowly. If you go slowly you're a lot more likely to take your time and do things right.

For instance, some of the sex tips are going to seem excessively clumsy for you. You'll try as much as possible to satisfy your partner. And the important part is that you're trying new things. You aren't letting your sex life stagnate. You're being adventurous and open to different experiences. That's the most telling sign of an **excellent lover.**

Now that you have the secrets, the next step is up to you. Don't flip through these pages and never pick up this book again! You must take the time and energy to put the sex secrets to work for you. Do so, and I promise, you'll enjoy it.

All the best,
Babalola Wasiu

About The Author

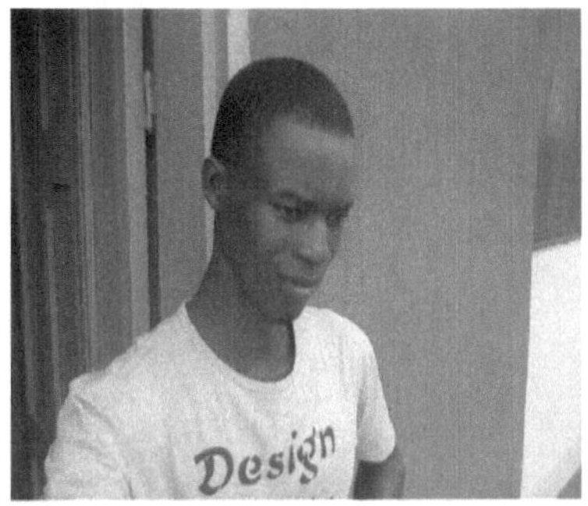

BABALOLA WASIU is the an Amazon book publisher author of _The Ultimate Instant Pot Cookbook_ and _Superfood Smoothies,_ among others. He lives in Osun State, Nigeria. Babalola Wasiu loves business, educating and inspiring other authors and entrepreneurs to succeed and live the life of their dreams.

Other Books By BABALOLA WASIU

The Ultimate Instant Pot Cookbook

Superfood Smoothies

11 Easy Ways to Get Clients

Sex Secrets

ONE LAST THING...

If you enjoyed this book or found it useful I'd be very grateful if you'd post a short review on Amazon. Your support really does make a difference and I read all the reviews personally so I can get your feedback and make this book even better.

Thanks again for your support!